PLEASE GET TO KNOW ME

AGING WITH DIGNITY AND RELEVANCE

PLEASE GET TO KNOW ME

VIRGINIA GARBERDING

WITH CECIL MURPHEY

Pleasant Word

A Division of WINEPRESS PUBLISHING

Pleasant Word (a division of WinePress Publishing, PO Box 428, Enumclaw, WA 98022) functions only as book publisher. As such, the ultimate design, content, editorial accuracy, and views expressed or implied in this work are those of the author.

ISBN 13: 978-1-4141-1207-7
ISBN 10: 1-4141-1207-6
Library of Congress Catalog Card Number: 2008901610

For the Reverend Martin C. Lopahs, who will always be with us in spirit, and Verona Lopahs, who continues to teach us how to live with grace, dignity, relevance, and as a witness, into our advanced years.

CONTENTS

ACKNOWLEDGMENT

Profound thanks to my very talented friends and colleagues Jeanne Heid-Grubman, Jennifer Bebinger, and Shari Floss, who have shared their knowledge, experience, and have encouraged me with their wise counsel and good humor. To Shari, my sage advisor, who coined the phrase many years ago, and hears the plea of the elderly to Please Get to Know Me.

To my sister Ruth Sazama, who has the talent to listen with unending enthusiasm, and to my daughters Beth, Karen, and Melissa, who always are my reason.

This book is written as a motivator for families to become an active member of the team taking care of their loved one. This book is in no way intended to take the place of professional legal or medical advice. The information presented is intended as a general guide; for specific guidance please refer to your local healthcare professionals.

INTRODUCTION: A LONG LIFE IS GOD'S GRACE

> Gray hair is a crown of glory; it is gained by living a godly life.
>
> (Prov. 16:31)

Who Am I and Why Am I Writing?

I'm writing this book from a double perspective. First, I'm writing this because I'm a registered nurse, certified in restorative nursing. For the last twenty plus years I have worked with the geriatric population as staff nurse and supervisor. During the last ten years, I've also worked as a nurse educator in a facility that specializes in persons with Alzheimer's disease or related dementias.

In these capacities I've been a member of the team at resident care conferences. Many times I've heard the frustrations of families as they try to be participants in their loved ones' care. I've comforted and counseled family members as they shared their feelings of dread at facing the nursing home visit.

I am currently Director of Education for staff and community at The Wealshire, which is located in Lincolnshire, Illinois. The Wealshire is a pioneering facility for the care of persons with Alzheimer's disease and related dementias.

Second, I'm writing this book because I've been the daughter of a nursing home resident for six years. This combination of being a nurse and a family member gives me a unique perspective on the issues of quality of care and quality of life. As a daughter, I've also felt the frustrations and feelings of helplessness that many family members experience as I viewed my mother's journey through admission and acclimation to acceptance. In this book, I move back and forth from being the professional facilitator to being the daughter of a parent in a nursing community.

All of the advances in public health have led us to a larger population of senior citizens than ever before. They are also the fastest growing segment of our population. The average life expectancy in the United States in 1900 was 47 years; today it is 77 years.

In the United States, we have begun to fear disability, both physical and cognitive, more than death. Who wants to be called old, elderly, or frail? Sometimes we need to have the meaning of frailty thrust upon us to feel empathy. For me, it was after many years of dramatic, painful episodes of disability related to arthritis. For months, I had to spend an enormous amount of time resting and using crutches to walk. By depending on my husband and daughter for many things, I grasped the idea of frailty. I needed help and had to depend on others.

During that time I also learned gratitude. I was grateful to God for the people who cared for me. I was grateful for the finances to support me without my having to worry. I was grateful to live at this time in history, when I had the medical and pharmaceutical means to care for me that hadn't been available even twenty-five years ago.

But most of all, I became grateful for the disability itself, and the way it forced me to slow down. The forced slowdown had unanticipated benefits and those results have lasted. I was forced to look inward and ponder where I had been, where I was, and to find inner strength for each day.

My pain and disability put me "in the moment," and I felt much like elders who can't predict the future. They hurt too much today to think about tomorrow or next week. I went inward and did the work that I wouldn't ordinarily have done if I hadn't been forced to make changes. Having the time to reminisce and to contemplate what had gone before without the distractions of a busy life changed me.

I learned many lessons and, in the process, I was able to see the needs of elders. For example, accumulation of things no longer matters. Elders are done with wanting things. Conceit and vanity over outward appearances are over. When our bodies begin to fail, we start to appreciate who we *are* and realize that we are much more than our appearance or ability to function.

I also understand why elders want their caregivers to see that they are much more than their needs. They want comfort, but comfort means relationships that are built around a kind word, or someone willing to spend time with them.

My disability helped me to realize that living in an atmosphere that focuses on elders and what is meaningful to them can be created in almost any environment. More and more elders are living in their own communities, often labeled as retirement centers. An ever-increasing number of elders or their families opt for the nursing home or nursing communities because of medical considerations or lack of family resources for caregiving.

It is unfortunate, but many people view going into a nursing home or skilled nursing facilities as just the time to mark before the end. They don't see that the community can also be a dignified environment to complete a life. Because of that sad perception, many elderly people fear nursing homes. Elders sometimes plead with their children, "Promise you will never put me in a nursing home."

So much stigma is attached to that concept of the old nursing facilities that smelled of urine, were often unclean, and elders often didn't receive proper care. Such places are now regulated by state and local laws. To stay open, they must be inspected regularly. Here are two suggestions.

1. **Don't promise you'll never place an elder in a nursing home.** You'll obviously mean the promise when you make it, but circumstances, such as the elder's deteriorating condition, may mean you can't keep that promise. Instead, say, "I promise to do what

I can to avoid putting you in a nursing home. If I have to put you in one, I'll put you in the best one possible, and I'll visit you as often as I can." (The promise to visit is important. Many elders feel they'll be abandoned once they go into a nursing home.)

2. **If you have promised and must go back on the promise, say to the elder, "I'm sorry."** Some elders may feel abandoned, neglected, or unloved if you have to go back on your promise. Keep as calm as possible and say, "I want you to have the best possible care. They can do for you what I can't, but I'll do what I can for you and I'll visit as often as I can."

I want to tell you about an elder named Hilda. She had been a synchronized swimmer in the Esther Williams movies of the 1940s. When she came to our facility she was in her eighties and was recovering from an infection. Hilda was still agile and could kick her foot over her head, which she was quite willing to demonstrate at any time.

Hilda had never married or had children; her attorney was her legal guardian. She lived in an affluent area west of Chicago in a large home with paid caregivers. She suffered from significant cognitive loss, but continued to be sociable and blossomed while she recuperated in the nursing community environment. She made friends, loved to go to activities, and especially loved our swimming pool. She wanted to live in our facility. However, the day came when she had to go back to her residence because of a promise her attorney had made to her: Years earlier he had promised, "I'll never let you be put into a nursing home."

"But I want to stay here," she insisted. I can only assume that he felt she wasn't able to make that decision. Despite Hilda's protests, he took her back to Chicago.

Elders living at home may still be restricted and have their life revolve around the tasks done for them. I once visited with a woman who lived in an apartment in a senior retirement community. Her son had lovingly provided a twenty-four hour caregiving service for her so that she could "stay in her home." However, after spending an afternoon with her and speaking to her son, I learned that she ate all her meals in her apartment. The other residents rejected her in the facility commons because she suffered serious memory impairment. Even though she had loved playing cards, taking walks, and watching musical videos (of which she owned many), she spent her days grooming, dressing, eating, and sitting on the couch with the caregiver. They watched soap operas and court TV all day.

Whatever place of residence is chosen, I want to offer information to empower family and friends so they can assist their loved ones in maintaining autonomy, individuality, and above all to continue to grow in Christian joy during their remaining years.

Chapter 1

COMMUNITY LIVING

> Then when you will call, the Lord will answer: "Yes, I am here," He will quickly reply.
>
> (Isa. 58:9)

Somewhere in our lives, most of us encounter the necessity of community living. We can look on those times with anticipation, excitement, joy, gratitude, and pride. It's much like an eighteen-year-old leaving for college after she has earned her place through academic achievement and parental financial sacrifice. However, entry into the nursing-home community is rarely met with excitement or happy anticipation. Elders seldom do it voluntarily.

Unlike the young college freshman, elders rarely anticipate the people they might meet, or relationships they'll form, or value the learning opportunities before them. The big difference is that elders don't move on to the next upward step in their careers. They don't see the community living as preparation for the next step in life or as a desirable stage of life. For elders, this is the final step. Just the idea of the *final* step can be depressing and disheartening. Or, it can become an invigorating climax to a well-lived life.

Community living may be the only option. Like college students, they have roommates, their own share of personal space, and get used to community shower rooms. They eat many times in cafeteria style off of a tray at a table with strangers. They can also make new friends and enjoy rich experiences.

Family members need to help elders focus positively on such a transition. Elders tend to see their entry into such communities as the end of a long line of experienced losses. They have lost homes and possessions accumulated over a lifetime. They've lost relationships and companionship through death, disability, and frailty, and they no longer have the challenge of learning and growing.

Through a lifetime of experience, many times elders have gone through the grieving process. The way in which they handled grief in the past can support them through this time of further loss and grieving. During times of grief and loss, the last thing they want is something new, and yet new seems to be all they have.

Many become angry or resentful. Those are normal reactions to grief. Along with that is the need to find someone or some organization to blame. It's usually safe to blame family members as they express their anger, resentment, and frustration. Elders are wise enough to realize that if they express their frustration toward the nursing staff they may be perceived as being difficult. Families can help new residents avoid being labeled as difficult. They can do that most effectively by taking an active role in the nursing community team.

When young people move into the academic community, it's time for the family to step back; however, it's the reverse here. During entrance into the nursing community elders need the family to step forward. The typical picture of elders in the nursing community is one of hopelessness and helplessness. Often the family feels much the same way.

Here are simple things to note and remember if you move an elder into a nursing facility.

1. **Let elders make as many decisions themselves as they can.** Allow them to do as much for themselves as possible. This is especially true for the cognitively intact individuals who must move into the nursing community out of medical necessity.

2. **Allow elders to feel their emotions and to express their sense of loss and grief.** Many times, a reassuring presence is what elders want and need. If friends and family express a quiet assurance and cooperation with the nursing staff, they make it easier for elders to adjust.

3. **Elders may feel confused and disoriented after they enter the community.** Be alert to that likelihood. They have the decreased ability to concentrate and yet have many unfamiliar faces to learn, a

new environment to adjust to, strange routines and schedules to adapt to. If your elder reacts with confusion, make certain the staff know this behavior is not typical.

4. **Take time to know those with whom your loved one will live.** In my case, I learned about the friends with whom Mom shared her life. One person is Rose, who has sat at her table in the dining room for the past year. At the time of this writing, Rose is 102, which makes her eighteen years older than Mom—old enough to be her mother. Rose can be quite a handful, and she tries Mom's patience. For instance, Rose likes to be the first one served and the first to leave for her nap. When she isn't first, she loudly complains that the members of the staff " . . . like the rest of you better than they like me."

   Even though Rose tells Mom every day, "You're the best friend I've ever had," if Mom goes first in anything, there will be trouble, and Rose will complain about Mom.

   When things seem to go sour for Rose, the first thing she does is declare, "This is hell." Mom seems constantly shocked at that declaration, even though it happens almost daily. Each time she informs Rose that they have good food and nice people to take care of them. "We're lucky to be here." That doesn't stop Rose from complaining

   "Rose, this is far from hell." Mom said one time in my presence. On that occasion Rose's pause gave

Mom the chance to talk about Jesus whom they both love.

One day I asked Mom, "Would you like to sit at another table so Rose won't bother you so much?"

"Oh no, I couldn't do that," she said. "Rose would think I've abandoned her."

I smiled and patted her check. It was exactly the right answer. Mom has chosen to remain Rose's best friend, regardless of the verbal abuse she endures. Interacting with her friend and having the opportunity to be supportive of another person empower Mom. They give her a wonderful thing—feeling strong and useful.

5. **Let elders talk.** They still experience life and they have things to talk about and to share. Let them. For example, Mom's closest friends are her direct caregivers and she tells me about them. During her more than six years at the facility, she has gotten close to them and likes them. They have little ongoing jokes with her, such as the nursing assistant who teases her, "I'm going to sell all of your china to finance my nursing education."

   "You will not! That is my china!" Mother asserts and they both laugh.

   On Sundays when I visit Mom, I don't want the conversation to be only about me and my life outside her community. I give her the chance to talk about what has happened during the past week and what she has done. Life goes on in the nursing home as well.

She often talks about the things they do during their activity classes. One week they studied mustard all week—the various types and where they come from. They were able to taste each of them. "I never knew there was so much to say about mustard," Mother said and smiled. She likes to learn new things; I like to have her tell me about them.

6. **Much of the adjustment to the nursing facility depends on the family.** How elders' families assist and support their loved one through education, encouragement, and understanding greatly determines their ability to say the famous Serenity Prayer: "God, grant me the serenity to accept the things I cannot change, courage to change the things I can, and the wisdom to know the difference."

CHAPTER 2

PLEASE GET TO KNOW ME

> [God said] "I knew you before I formed you in your mother's womb. Before you were born I set you apart and appointed you as my spokesman to the world."
>
> (Jer. 1:5)

Mabel died today. Minutes later, a nurse hurried down the hall carrying two old books. She stopped and excitedly showed me what the staff found when they cleaned Mabel's room. She held up books on physics. "Mabel wrote them! Can you believe that? I never knew she wrote anything."

We had cared for Mabel for six years, but none of us staff knew she had written any books. When she came to us, Mabel was already afflicted with Alzheimer's disease. We learned later that Mabel had been a prominent physicist.

As I listened to the nurse, I thought, *Wouldn't it have been wonderful if Mabel could have enjoyed our expressions of respect, awe, and admiration?* Now it was too late.

That true story isn't an isolated instance. Too often the nursing home staff learns information about residents from reading the obituaries. The individual life stories never make it to the direct care staff, even if it had been reported to social workers on admission. The story had been diluted to minimum facts on a fill-in sheet at the back of the chart under the Social Service tab.

With the focus on patient confidentiality, the direct caregivers have access only to the information needed so they can do their jobs. They receive information such as whether the elders are continent, whether they can brush their teeth, bathe independently, or need walkers.

For quality of life, the information needed by the staff involves such things as who they are and something about their families, where they came from, and what they've accomplished in their lives. As it is now in the admission interviews, the conversations between family and caregivers revolve around the tasks of caring for the elder.

Too often the individuals become known only by their diagnosis. The new hip in 403, the Parkinson's in 602, or the hip replacement in 403—instead of Mrs. Jones in 403. I became sensitive to that need early in my nursing career, when I took care of an elderly man with Alzheimer's disease. His children had handwritten a letter to the staff and it was posted on his door. It began with these words: "Dad worked his entire life with cardboard."

Their father started his own company, and they told about the cardboard products he had produced. They provided a list of topics on which he could still converse. They even posed questions that dealt with his passion for cardboard.

They gave their father a beautiful gift, but that gift was also for his caregivers. That short message had the power to give back to their father an important part of his life—an opportunity to remember his accomplishments by giving to his caregivers the tools for a meaningful connection.

During times of routine daily care, instead of talking about the task at hand—or even worse, not speaking—and giving the man no feelings of connection with his caregivers, all staff members had information to make a connection with him. They could see him as a husband, father, manufacturer, *and* as a person.

That single incident helped me to realize the importance of family and friends sharing the life story of their loved ones. By having direct caregiver information, the staff can provide better care.

For instance, if we know that the man has four daughters, that information could prompt caregivers to say that they also have daughters. They can discuss the joys and the heartaches of raising their children. Just that small piece of information can create a connection between caregivers and elders. As caregivers learn more about the individuals, they have more opportunity to give more of themselves, and the elders want a connection with their caregivers.

By providing that personal information, families empower the caregivers. Information enables caregivers to move from the impersonal to the personal. When families provide information, they give the hip replacement woman a name and an identity.

For example, a regular nurse might tell a float-caregiver, "Oh, you have Mary today. Did you know that Mary was a kindergarten teacher for forty-five years?" Such information creates an immediate reaction in how the caregiver perceives Mary. The caregiver sees not just an elderly woman who is nonverbal and needs total care, but someone who was a dedicated teacher and role model to young children for many years.

Here's an example from my own life. My mother's brother, Ed, once took a bicycle trip across the country. He traveled coast to coast, taking odd jobs to pay his expenses. When he was in his late seventies, his wife died. Uncle Ed was diagnosed with Alzheimer's, and my mother became his legal guardian. When Uncle Ed needed an assisted-living facility, mother wrote a short biography of his life and his lifelong interest in cycling. She also provided him with a bicycle.

As Uncle Ed's disease progressed, he went from assisted living to total care. But during his journey through Alzheimer's disease, his passion for cycling was supported by an informed staff. He began with independent biking around the neighborhood to having a nursing assistant accompany him on another bike, and finally he had a stationary bike in his room with a nursing assistant's support. By letting the staff know how important that exercise was to Uncle

Ed, we were able to empower the staff and temporarily give back to Uncle Ed the life he was forgetting.

Instead of a life only of being kept clean, dry, fed, and visitor-ready, the knowledge of his interest created conversation and encouraged the staff to think creatively of ways to enable him to continue his interest until his last days.

Here's another way to provide information. When my mother was admitted to the nursing facility, every two or three weeks I posted a new note on her closet door titled, "Please Get To Know Me." I chose paper with a border of forget-me-nots for my notes. This week I left the following:

PLEASE GET TO KNOW ME

Verona is an artist and specialized in china painting. She took her first art class in her early forties and enjoyed more than forty years of china painting. Over those years she produced a large amount of work, including hand-painted tea sets for each of her fifteen grandchildren. Each one received the china as a wedding present. She painted every piece in her china cabinet.

Although her corner china cabinet had been with her since she entered the nursing facility, Mother told me that after reading the posted note, the staff took time to look at the items in the cabinet. They talked to her about her career as an artist.

Here are two other notes I posted:

Please Get to Know Me

Verona liked math in school. After she married Martin, a Lutheran minister, she took over the family finances. For many years the family income was less than $10,000. From that salary, they supported a family of six. Verona shopped only twice a month for groceries and they gave ten per cent to the church and were able to educate their children.

They never had more than one charge account and paid it off quickly when they used it. They never owned more than one car at a time. Verona budgeted money for vacations and retirement.

Please Get to Know Me

Verona loved her class in religion in high school and married Martin, a Lutheran minister. They were married for sixty-two years and served congregations in Texas, Illinois, and Wisconsin. Verona enjoys talking about Jesus and her favorite topic of heaven.

Please support Verona's faith by turning on her Christian radio station for her when she is in bed.

I keep the notes brief and recycle them occasionally for the benefit of new staff members. Mother told me that after I put up the signs, female caregivers spoke with her and several sought her advice. One frequent question she received was, "How do you find a good man?" Another was, "What is the secret of such a long marriage?"

An opportunity to counsel struggling single mothers encourages Mother. To know that her advice is wanted and appreciated means so much to her. Those conversations give her a chance to witness of her faith to her caregivers—people she wouldn't have the opportunity to meet if she weren't in a nursing community.

There are other ways to help the staff know elders. Some families post pictures of the loved ones participating in areas of special interest. A picture of Dad golfing, or Mom riding a horse, can prompt conversation with even a nonverbal person. "Mabel, is that you on the horse?"

A short note stating that Mabel is a great-grandmother can lead the caregiver to the overlooked pictures on the wall with, "Oh, Mabel, are these your great-grandchildren over here?"

Mementos of an exciting career are another helpful thing, especially if there is a note of explanation. At one facility where I worked, we observed Veteran's Day and recognized residents who had served in the armed services.

I still remember a picture of a resident standing next to General Douglas MacArthur, with whom he had served. Even though the man had been a resident for several years, I looked at him a little differently after having had that glimpse into his life.

I'm convinced that any opportunity to provide a link with who they are, where they came from, what they have done, and what they would like to be remembered for can prompt personal conversation. That leads away from conversation about the task at hand and promotes a higher quality of life for elders, while providing the comfort of living with those who know them.

Chapter 3

"M" IS FOR THE MANY THINGS SHE GAVE ME

What is the price of five sparrows? A couple of pennies? Yet God does not forget a single one of them. And the very hairs on your head are all numbered. So don't be afraid; you are more valuable to him than a whole flock of sparrows.

(Luke 12:6-7)

"Sometimes I feel invisible," my mother said as she looked into the face of her nurse.

"Oh, honey, sometimes we all feel invisible," the nurse said as she patted my mother's hand in what I considered a condescending manner. "Now just take your pills." Immediately, she hurried off to other residents.

"What did you mean by feeling invisible?" I asked my mother.

"When I call to a nurse for anything—a tissue, a drink, or to go to the bathroom—they walk past me as if I don't exist, as if I'm invisible."

"How does that make you feel when they pretend they don't hear you?"

After a pause, she said, "Sad. Just sad."

As I sat beside her, I thought of the woman who dozed in her wheelchair. She was my mother. When I was a child, I called her "Mommy." For many years thereafter, it was "Mom." As the years have gone by for my siblings and me, we began to call her Mother, as though we knew the time was short. Too soon we will no longer have that person who has been so central in each of our lives.

"Mother," I whispered aloud. I don't think she heard me.

As I contemplated how much she meant to me, I remembered a poem I sent to one of my daughters on her first Mother's Day as a new mother. The poem told of a baby soon to be born. God told the baby not to be afraid because someone would be there. The baby asked, "How will I know her? What is her name"

"You will call her Mother," God said.

As I reflected on those words, I gazed at my eighty-four-year-old mother in her wheelchair and wondered how I could help the nursing staff to see her, and to also help her move beyond feeling helpless and hopeless. I assumed that residents of other nursing communities felt the same way.

I smiled as I remembered when a close friend explained the difference between a new purchase of a costly picture and a nursing-community resident. Often when we purchase something new for our home such as a prized picture, we pick exactly the right spot for it, and we know it will look beautiful in that special place. For a period of time, we enjoy it; however, after awhile we no longer notice it unless someone calls our attention to it. That reminds us how much we like that picture.

The more I thought about it, the more I believed it was a fair analogy. Staff members who don't respond when residents call out may have become desensitized. They might be kind caregivers and sincerely care about the elders, but not everyone can maintain a high awareness day after day, feel and express empathy, and "see" those for whom they care.

The nursing community staff is highly task oriented. For example, nurses are concerned with how many medications they have to give within the state guidelines to provide medication within one hour of the time designated. Along with that, they have other tasks that they have to do, including charting. It's easy and perhaps natural for them to focus only on the immediate task.

Besides that, each shift has its own set of duties. Nursing assistants have to get people up for the day. That means washing the incontinent, as well as dressing, combing hair, washing faces, brushing teeth, and many times transferring residents into wheelchairs.

After residents are up, nursing assistants have to straighten up the rooms. During meal times, they bring their residents to the dining room, serve them their meals, and assist residents by opening containers, cutting food, seating those residents who can eat independently, and providing total assistance to those no longer able to eat independently.

Because of so many demands on the staff, many residents, like my mother, become invisible. After a period of time the caregivers no longer see the elders or hear them even though they may truly care.

That brought up a serious question for me: How do the family members assist the staff to see, and continue to see?

Chapter 4

CREATE A BUZZ

> God blesses the people who patiently endure testing. Afterward they will receive the crown of life that God has promised to those who love him.
>
> (James 1:12)

It started with the cookbook. Mother had been in a nursing community for about three years after her stroke, and Dad had an apartment in another area of the Christian complex. Christmas was coming and I asked Mother if she would like me to copy some of her recipes. I agreed to put them into book form for Christmas gifts to her grandchildren. Many of the recipes had come from Germany with the family.

Once we decided to do the cookbook together, she, Dad, and I spent many Sunday afternoons to choose what would be included. Those were also nostalgic times, as we reminisced about occasions when we had used those recipes.

My youngest daughter, Missy, started going to the nursing home with me. We decided that when we were ready, Missy would write and assemble the book. Dad contributed comments or witticisms, such as, "We always called this 'enthusiastic stew,' because we threw everything we had into it."

To further stimulate our gastric juices, several times I cooked one of those dishes, brought it for my Sunday visit, and heated it in Dad's oven. Those days of remembering food and special times created many poignant memories I carry today.

Two months later, when we had accomplished our purpose, Missy and I brought in twenty copies of the book. My parents signed a book for each child and grandchild, wrapped them, and had them ready for Christmas. We left one copy on Mother's bedside table so that she could look at it whenever she liked.

That's when it started—with a cookbook. We had no idea that it would affect the staff. After that, whenever I visited, staff members from various departments approached me and requested a copy. I gladly brought them copies, because it was an opportunity to bring Mother out of the shadows and to introduce her to the staff as an excellent cook. They loved to talk to Mother about cooking, and I saw new light shining in her eyes.

I frequently cooked and brought in some of her specialties, and also included several copies of the recipe from Mother's cookbook. When I brought in brown coffee cake, our family's favorite, I placed the cake and the recipe in the employee kitchen with a note from Mother, telling them to eat and enjoy the cake.

That simple thing made such a difference. The nursing staff, activity staff, and housekeepers stopped by mother's room to tell her how much they enjoyed her coffee cake and thanked her for the recipe. The pleasure on my mother's face was worth all the effort we had put into the book and the cooking. I tell this story because it taught me the importance of family and friends connecting the elder to the staff that cares for our loved ones.

The connection can be simple. For example, include the elder in conversations. When the family converses with staff, they can make it their practice to be with their loved one and to defer to him or her. Let her speak and explain her preferences.

Another thing: the simple gesture of squatting beside a person in a wheelchair provides direct eye contact and reminds us to include that person in our conversations.

Common introductions are often not observed in the nursing community. Here's an easy way to change that. Whenever family members bring the elder into the dining room, one of them can take the initiative and say, "Hello, I'm Shirley and this is my mother, Ruth Smith. Ruth just moved in yesterday. I see they are having meatloaf today for lunch. Ruth was known for her meatloaf at church potlucks."

I've been aware that most nursing community dining rooms are filled with conversation about how much everyone ate or should eat. "Come on, Mabel, just one more bite." Why not make it a good experience? We can inject social conversation that makes a quality dining experience. When we visit, we can

- stimulate the conversation
- ask questions
- make observations
- pay attention to those around your loved one
- get the names of the others and remember them.

It's not that difficult to make the dining room a pleasant place to be. Just such simple social interactions benefit not only our loved one, but the other residents within hearing distance. I once observed Edith, the caring wife of a former Chicago Cubs baseball player. Tom had advanced Alzheimer's disease and was no longer verbal. Edith provided numerous Cubs caps and shirts so Tom could show his support of the team. She made certain that Tom never missed a televised game. When Edith wasn't able to be with Tom herself, she phoned the staff and told them when the game was on and they made certain Tom could watch it.

On opening day of the baseball season, Edith brought in baseball-decorated cupcakes for everyone, so they could celebrate with Tom. When she visited with Tom and anyone came around, she shared information about the Cubs' standing in the league. The expression of happiness and connection on Tom's face is something I can't forget.

I loved to watch them sit together. His Alzheimer's was so advanced, it was obvious he didn't understand the various plays, but that didn't matter. Most of the time, Tom stroked his glove as he focused on the TV. Because of Edith's ongoing efforts, she kept Tom engaged in his former way of life until he died.

It takes so little to help loved ones connect with the world around them. Here are some of the ways I supported my mother's interests and life experiences.

Connection with the Community

After God called Dad home, we realized that Mother needed our help to remain connected to her friends, extended family, and Christian community. My sister and I determined to maintain Mother's Christmas card list. As a kind of family activity, we addressed the Christmas cards with Mother and mailed them Thanksgiving weekend. By sending them early, everyone would have her current address in the nursing facility, and could add her to their Christmas list. That Christmas, she received more than sixty cards, which amazed the staff. It also made them aware that many people outside the nursing facility thought of and cared about that elderly nursing home resident.

The Artist

What followed was a show-and-tell event by one of my sisters. After asking the director's permission, my sister brought samples of Mother's forty-plus years of china painting. She brought a tea set, Christmas plates, ornaments, piggy banks, and crosses—all hand-painted by Mother. That presentation interested other residents as well as the nursing and activity staff. Mother was officially recognized in the facility as the artist that she is.

Her Car

When Mother first came to the nursing facility, she was able to drive an electric wheelchair. Because Dad was no longer able to drive, we took the license plate from their Buick and attached it to the back of Mother's wheelchair and put her still-current driver's license in her purse. That turned out to be a great way for her to get acquainted. Staff and residents saw the license plate and asked, "Hey, do you have a license to drive that thing?"

With twinkling eyes, Mother proudly produced her driver's license. She enjoyed the attention, met a lot of people, and never tired of the joke.

Grooming

Even the small day-to-day things can mean so much. Mother liked to wear colored beads every day with her outfits. We couldn't expect the nursing assistants to keep track of her jewelry, so we installed removable adhesive hooks to the inside of her closet door and hung multiple strands of colored beads within easy reach. Mother has a standard outfit of black pants and a white or black cardigan sweater that she wears with a bright colored top and a string of beads every day. The system proved successful because staff members no longer had to try to coordinate her clothes. Mother is happy. The staff is happy because we haven't tried to add any additional duties for them. They can easily help her put an outfit together and it creates less stress for everyone involved.

A standing appointment in the beauty parlor every Friday helps Mother keep track of the days in the week and provides an additional opportunity to visit with other people and make more acquaintances. Mother has a simple, short, and curly hairdo. Each Sunday afternoon, I reorganize Mother's closet as well as straighten up her room as part of her care team.

Changing Mother's clothes seasonally and taking them home to store, as well as bringing in special seasonal outfits like her black velvet pants suit, keeps her and the staff interested in her appearance. When Mother needs new clothes, I bring in catalogs and we make an occasion out of shopping.

The Birds

Mother liked birds and collected pictures of different species to include in her china painting. We decided to put a hummingbird feeder just outside her bedroom window to attract the lively little birds. The addition of long, flowing red ribbons aided in attracting the tiny visitors. We attached red and yellow gel hearts to the window, and it makes a pleasant view. The view not only pleases Mother, but lightens the mood of the most stoic caregiver and the occasional visitor. When staff members come into her room for the required hands-on care, they often see the tiny little birds perched on the feeder.

The sight creates immediate conversation between Mother and her caregiver. They share knowledge of birds, memories of past experiences with animals, the love of nature, or something that enables the caregiver to get to know Mother better. When visitors walk down the corridor and casually glance into Mother's room and see the tiny birds feeding, it often draws them into Mother's room to socialize with her.

Her Life Story

Because she had had a stroke, we knew Mother could no longer hold her photo albums. She was also in a wheelchair and couldn't get to them without help. Once I realized the situation, I took photos out of her albums and Missy scanned them on her computer. We added piano music of the big-band era and created Mother's own set of reminiscing DVDs.

Each of the DVDs lasts about forty-five minutes and we spaced the photos fifteen seconds apart. That gives her time to focus on them and reminisce.

"That's perfect," Mother said.

The nursing assistants have become knowledgeable about Mother's life because they sometimes join her in watching the DVDs. They see the progress of her life from being a child, to a teenager, and to being newly engaged. They often linger over her wedding pictures, and the DVD continues on through raising her children. Seeing Mother as young, and her life played out in pictures, provides conversation with her caregivers while it helps her stay in touch with her life story.

When the Stars Shine at Night

Dad had no interest in decorating. For him, anything that Mother liked was fine. But in his later years, no matter where they moved, he had a grandchild move his glow-in-the-dark stars of various sizes. For each move, the stars would have to be taken down and re-assembled. He kept them on the ceiling of his bedroom in the shape of a cross. After Dad got ready for bed and turned off the lights, the last thing he saw before he drifted off was the star cross.

Even though Dad is gone, we continue the tradition over Mother's bed. This has impacted the staff and brought comfort to Mother. It also brings comfort to us because we know that the last thing she sees before she falls asleep is the cross.

Spending the time and thinking through the areas that gave meaning to the elder's life will reap rewards. When Tom's wife made the effort to let everyone know who Tom was, she validated his life for him as well as his caregivers. Seeing, reading, and sometimes tasting the results of Mom's cookbook validates her as the cook she was.

Being attentive to her clothes and maintaining Mom's hairstyle validates for her who she is every time she looks into the mirror. The old and very old need validation of who they are, just as we all do.

Chapter 5

COME IN—THE DOOR'S OPEN

Keep on asking, and you will receive what you ask for. Keep on knocking, and the door will be opened to you.
(Matt. 7:7)

For the many years after I was married and raising children, going to visit Mom and Dad was a little retreat. They were about an hour's drive away. When I arrived, I could expect to hear Mom calling out when we came to the door, "Come on in. The door is open."

Mom would stand inside the kitchen where the coffee would be on. I counted on something ready to munch on immediately, because we had just driven for a full hour, and she was ready for us. After that, Mom had a meal planned around something she knew I enjoyed.

Those visits involved sitting around the kitchen table eating, drinking, and talking. Their apartment would have ample reading material. Dad read only the Bible, the daily paper, and a few Christian periodicals. Besides her Bible, Mom read magazines and books on health and art. Our conversations revolved around news, politics, sports, health, Mom's art, and catching up on family news. We frequently played cards or sang together.

It was a mini-retreat for me because Mom provided excellent food, and Dad looked forward to feeding babies and playing with grandchildren. For those few hours, I relaxed and let them take over. It was sweet, and even now, years later, I miss those times together.

After Mom's stroke and entry into the nursing community, the quality of the visits was up to me. If there was any food, I was the one who provided it. I introduced news and family information. I had become the one who brought the outside world and community into their world.

The visit could have easily revolved around Mom's condition and a critique of her care, but how would that constitute a real visit? It was up to me to create the right kind of atmosphere so Mom would feel better when I left and could say, "We had such a good visit."

I write this because of the many times I've observed families who came to see their mom or grandma standing around awkwardly for twenty or thirty minutes, and focused almost entirely in talking about how she looked. After that they seemed to have run out of words, and they left shortly afterward. Or sometimes family and friends stood back and watched the staff activity of running a nursing community, as if they were intruders or observers of something quite important. They didn't seem to realize that the important thing was their visit to the elder. Nothing else was significant.

I thought of the flurry of activity and energy when I was a child when Mom prepared everything for our visits to Grandma's house. It was important to Mom; it was important to Grandma. I decided I needed to plan and have things ready for a memorable visit to my mother.

A good visit involved some serious planning by either having things readily available in the elder's room or brought in for a particular visit. We brought in our own folding chairs and kept them next to her closet to provide seating for several people. We kept playing cards and her address book in a drawer so we had a game to play, or we might call one of her friends to join us. We scouted the facility for little-used areas, such as the game room, where we sat around a table and played cards or simply talked. Often, we went to a piano when no one else was playing. We gathered around and my sister, Ruth, played songs we all knew. It was delightful to sing together.

We couldn't claim any space as "our place." At times we had to be flexible and move to accommodate other elders and their families.

Suggestions for Visits

1. **Keep in touch with the elder through correspondence or telephone.** Many times their going into a nursing community means the elder breaking ties with their longtime friends. That's when the family can step in and bridge that gap of keeping in touch.

- They can send cards or make phone calls.
- They can ask friends or other family members to keep the elder connected by mailing cards and pictures.
- They can ask the church to send the Sunday bulletin and monthly newsletter. If necessary, family members can read it to the elder during visits.

2. **Observe religious holidays with appropriate food and decorations.**

- Make this a time to talk about holiday foods in their season.
- Bring pictures and reminisce about wonderful family holidays.
- Have the elder's grandchildren make Christmas cookies. Bring them into the nursing home so Grandma can help decorate the cookies.
- Bring in the elder's long-collected decorations and make the room look festive to fit the season.
- Go to a craft store and buy a small Christmas tree to hang on a wall. (When cords are plugged in behind furniture, remote switches work well).
- Bring in an Easter lily or a pumpkin and colored paper for Thanksgiving.
- Munch on donuts and sip hot chocolate.
- Bring in your family's traditions and turn on the CD player and play Christmas carols.

3. **Enjoy a family-prepared meal together.** Much of the enjoyment of a good meal comes from the preparation and anticipation of it. If you plan to cook and bring something special to the nursing home, call your elder. Let that person experience the joy of anticipation. It becomes more than just the matter of eating the food.

   If possible, bring in cold ingredients and make a family favorite dish together at the nursing community. Let the elder experience the pleasure of cooking by mixing the ingredients and cooking the meal. Many times, food is one of the last remaining pleasures. Talk about such meals, plan for them, and make every visit special by bringing in some food the elder likes.

4. **Go outside.** Many elders in nursing communities no longer have the opportunity to go outside. Seek out quiet outdoor areas to visit, even if it's only feet away from the door. For them to be in natural air and light will be worth the effort you go through.

5. **Tour the facility.**

   - Walk through the facility and make yourself the official greeting committee.
   - Greet people and introduce your resident.
   - Find a place where you can sit and visit. Invite other families to join you.

- When you introduce your elder, add personal information that gives the elder an opportunity to remember a special accomplishment or pleasant memory.
- Steer the conversation away from a critique of the nursing community, staff, or food. (You want to support the elder's confidence in the staff, as well as the facility. Negative observations can be shared with the appropriate department at another time. Remember that even an elder suffering from dementia is sensitive to tone of voice and body language.)

6. **Work on a life story book together.** Gather memorabilia from your elder's life story. A three-ring binder works well with any type of stiff poster paper that can survive frequent handling. Be sure to include:

    - key life events, as well as copies of awards and certificates.
    - maps of places the elder has been.
    - work and armed service history.
    - add a family tree and indicate relationships to the elder.

By looking at the life story book with the elder, you give the staff the opportunity to appreciate the elder's life. When a staff member learns that a totally dependent elder is one who has had an extensive education or enjoyed a wonderful career or held a meaningful place in the community, it can promote increased care with dignity.

Elders will usually get excited and involved when told, "Let's work on your story book for the grandchildren." Having a project to work on for their children or grandchildren gives back to the elder the pleasure of being a grandparent or great-grandparent.

7. **Tips for when the elder is a man.**

- Watch a DVD (on travel, sports, history—whatever the man likes).
- Bring in something connected to his past interest to provide a comfortable visit.
- Read sports magazines together or critique new car brochures. Both are excellent opportunities for great conversations.
- Most men like to do something physical. Do that but keep it simple. Toss a ball or throw bean bags. Such activities can also effectively involve children with the elder.
- Watching funny DVDs together can be an especially wonderful connection for a son with his father.

My father-in-law suffered from dementia. My husband, Jerry, knew his dad had enjoyed Laurel and Hardy films as well as those of Ma and Pa Kettle—the comedies of the 1930s and 1940s. Jerry found as many of those old movies as he could and brought them to the nursing home. On his visits, Jerry didn't have to carry on long one-sided conversations.

When Jerry visited, he would tell his dad what was new with him and the family. After that, he put on an old movie and his dad laughed every time Jerry would laugh. We never knew how much he followed the story, or even "saw" the slap-stick comedy. But he could still enjoy that comfortable, normal activity of sitting with his son and laughing.

8. **Invite old friends, as well as members of clubs and organizations, to visit.** Much of the enjoyment of an occasion comes from planning it. Involve the elder in picking out the invitations, addressing the invitations, deciding on the refreshments, choosing clothes to wear—all the details that the elder would have done when hosting an occasion in the past.

   Ask those at the facility what arrangements could be made with the kitchen for visitors' meals and what areas you could use for private parties. Many times those areas have to be reserved, especially during holidays.

9. **Play card and board games.**

   - Bring cards to the facility and keep them in the elder's room.
   - Even if the elder can no longer actively participate in the game, just being in the room and

hearing family members play and laugh can be comforting.

- Have cards and board games available to occupy children and provide a pleasant memory for them of visiting Grandma or Grandpa.
- A lively game of Old Maid can be easy for the elder as well as a young child.

10. **Be ready to change plans.** Be aware that in a nursing community things can change quickly. For example, you settle down to read to Mom and the nursing assistant brings in her roommate, who doesn't feel well and wants to go to bed. That means you'll have to leave the room.

    Be ready to adapt. That could be a good time for a walk. You might also find a quiet spot to enjoy reading to the elder.

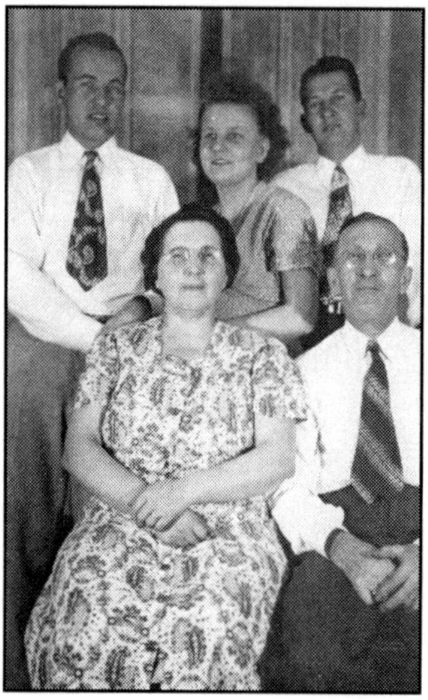

Verona with her parents and brothers Ed and Harvey – 1940

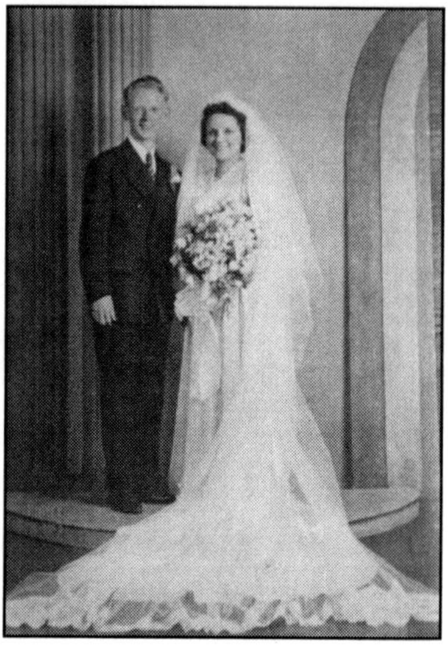

Verona and Martin June 19, 1943

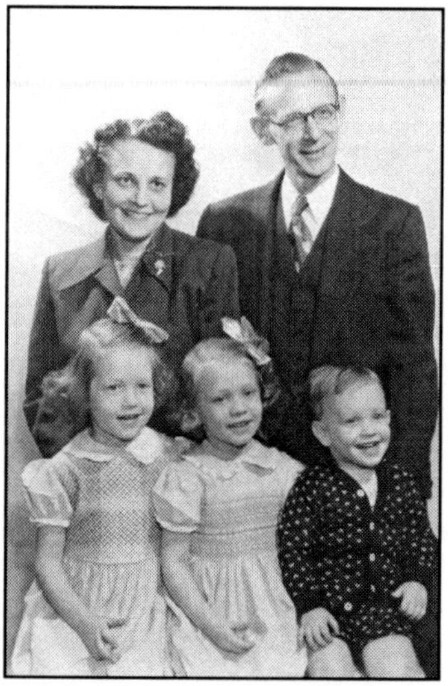

The Pastor's family – Ruth, Virginia, and Marty – 1952

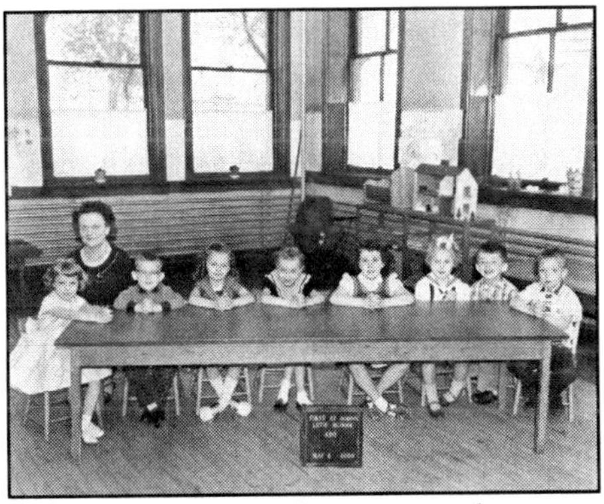

Verona the kindergarten teacher

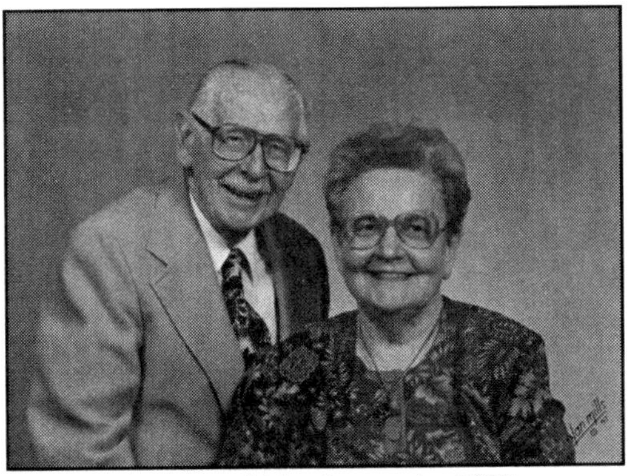

Verona and Martin – retire 1983

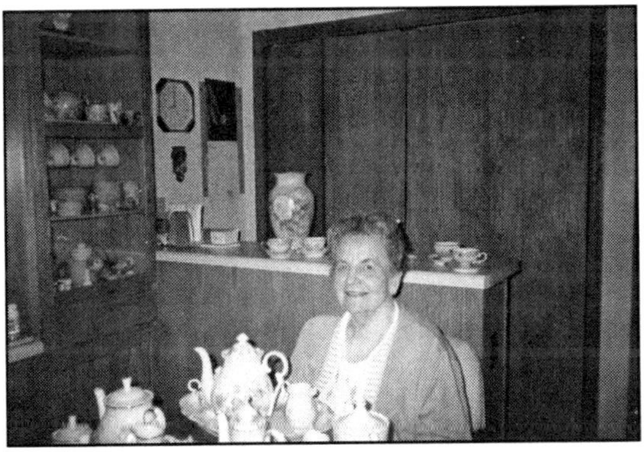

Verona the artist with her china

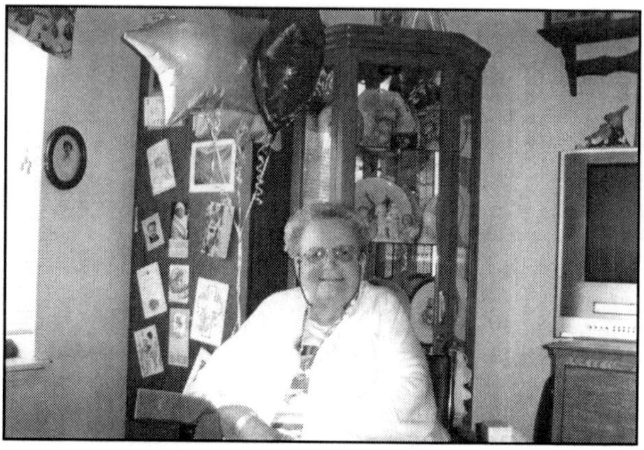

Verona's 84th birthday in the nursing home

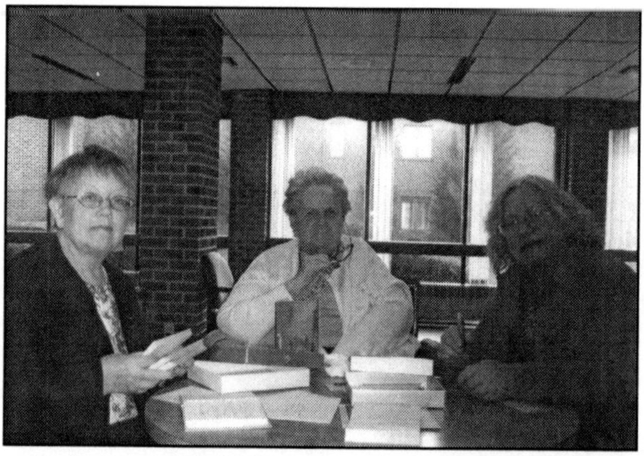

Ruth, Verona, and Virginia send out Christmas cards

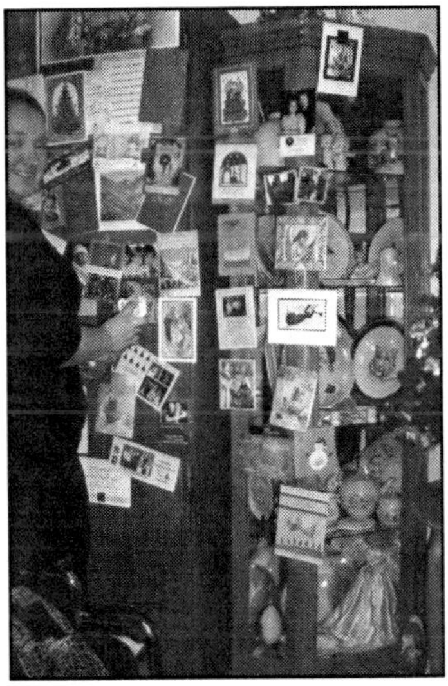

Missy decorates with Verona's
Christmas cards – 2007

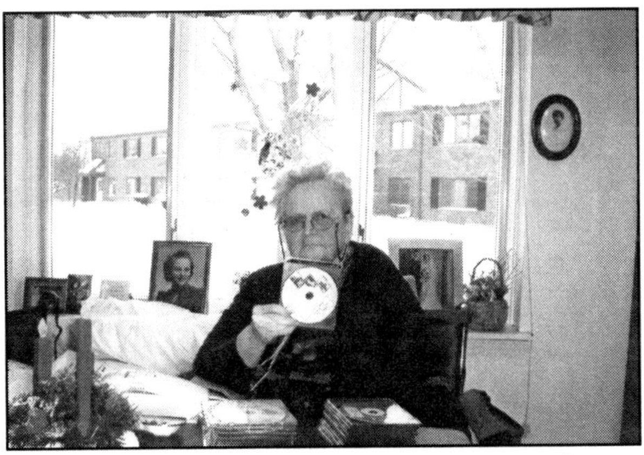

Verona with her twenty DVDS of her pictures that
she is giving family for Christmas 2007

Chapter 6

THE BEST-LAID PLANS

> Dear brothers and sisters, when troubles come your way, consider it an opportunity for great joy. For you know that when your faith is tested, your endurance has a chance to grow.
>
> (James 1:2-3)

Communication, communication, communication. We say it all the time, yet how do we follow through?

"It" started on a Friday afternoon. My sister Ruth and I went to the nursing community to visit Mother and inform the staff of our upcoming festivities. My three daughters would visit Saturday evening with their families and we'd take Mother out in a van to a local supper club. We had made arrangements that included an on-site inspection of local eateries, assessed noise levels, handicap accessibility, and width of aisles between tables for ease of wheelchair maneuvering. We checked menu offerings and sampled their food before we chose the site. We were almost ready.

The night before, we selected Mom's clothes and hung them outside her closet door so we could pick her up Saturday evening. We crossed off all the to-do items, and the only thing left to do was to notify the staff that we would take Mother. Everyone knew.

Saturday morning we went back to the nursing community for a final run-through of the evening plans. Mother was dressed in the chosen clothes, but at breakfast, she spilled food all over the front of her outfit. We checked her closet and found a new outfit. Again, we notified the staff by speaking directly with each caregiver as well as the nurse. "Please pass this information on to the evening shift," I said. I pointed out the new clothing we had hung outside of her closet.

"Yes, we'll do that," the supervisor assured me.

While Mother took an afternoon nap, we went to our hotel. We felt such a sense of relief: Everything was ready. Just to make sure, we arrived at the nursing community an hour earlier than planned. There sat Mother, up early from her nap and re-dressed in her breakfast encrusted clothes. I notified the nursing assistants, "Mother is going out with the family for dinner."

They were busily working with Mother's roommate, Harriett. The assistant looked up at me and said, "No one told us. Besides, Harriet is also going out. She has her rights, too."

"Of course Harriet has rights," I said. "And so does my mother." I calmed down and one assistant turned to my mother and, with her fingernail, scraped at the stained food. "Do you want to be changed, Verona?"

Before mother could answer, I knew where the conversation was headed. If she said no, the assistant would insist, "If she doesn't want to be changed, she doesn't have to change." She might also remind me of my mother's rights.

The matter of rights is like the proverbial two-edged sword, and the staff can be savvy in using it. If the nurse or assistant stands over a resident and uses a tone that indicates wanting and agreement, the elder can be easily intimidated into cooperating with the staff.

"Do you want to be changed?" the assistant asked again.

"Yes, I want to change," Mother said, to my surprise.

"We will get back to you when we have time," the nursing assistant answered. I raced from the room and found the PM nurse. I implored her to intervene. Together we went back to Mother's room and she told the assistant, "Please take care of Verona."

The assistant nodded and grudgingly accommodated the request. As soon as she had done the minimal amount, she again turned her attention to Harriet.

I had to comb Mother's hair, put her jewelry on her, wash her glasses, and get out a sweater for her to wear—things the assistant should have already done.

I sighed, thinking that everything was ready. That's when I realized we had a problem with the wheelchair. Mother uses an electric one, but it's too large for the van, so she would have to go in her manual chair. Her manual chair was missing.

I raised a fuss and asked several assistants. One of them finally said sheepishly, "Yes, now I remember. Yesterday they needed a wheelchair for a new resident. Your mother never uses hers, so they borrowed it." (I noticed it was "they" who did such things.)

I took several deep breaths and searched the facility, but we couldn't find Mother's chair. I finally realized that unless we could get the electric wheelchair on the ramps, mother would not be able to go to dinner with us.

Just about then, the pampered and coiffed Harriett came out of the room. She looked as if she was a member of a wedding party with a gold lame' jacket and jewelry. Her make-up was flawless. When the assistant wheeled her down to the sitting room, she called out, "Here's Harriet."

No one moved. Twelve people sat in the room. All of them were there for my mother. Minutes later, the van arrived and, with quite a bit of difficulty, we were able to get Mother's electric chair onto the ramp.

Just before we left, I overheard the nursing assistant's telephone call to Harriet's daughter. "Your mother is ready. Where are you?" I stood there and unashamedly listened. The next words I heard were, "What do you mean 'she isn't going out'?" She told the daughter to hold on while she checked.

The nurse who checked said, "131-A is going out with the family at 4:30 p.m. 131-B isn't going anywhere." My mother was 131-A.

The assistant received the bad news: Ninety-year-old, hard-of-hearing Harriet was not going out. She wheeled Harriet back to her room.

How do those things happen? Is it only a one-time experience? I wish I could answer yes, but that would not be true. Such things happen a lot more often than the staff would like to acknowledge. For one thing, the staff changes every eight hours. Verbal requests often get forgotten or remembered incorrectly.

It makes me think of the children's game called "Telephone" where they form a circle. The leader whispers to the first person, who whispers it to the next. The last child repeats the message heard. In almost every instance, the final message is nothing like the original.

In this account, the only way to improve on that communication would have been with an excessive amount of writing. I could have started with a memo to the nurses to put every bit of the information on their 24-hour clipboard, along with my contact number. I would have followed up with longer notes to the staff written on colored paper and posted strategically around the room. I would also have had to have a large sign hanging on the coat hanger with the clothes, and again write out all the information about every item Mother would wear, and include my contact number.

Post-it notes don't work. They have to be large and fully informative. That's still not the end. I would have had to follow through with phone calls and last minute double on-site checking.

Think of the communication this way: When the family counts on only verbal communication, the vital information just walks out the door with the last shift.

Chapter 7

COMMUNICATION

> Trust in the Lord with all your heart; do not depend on your own understanding. Seek his will in all you do, and he will show you which path to take.
>
> (Prov. 3:5-6)

Family members aren't always the recognized authorities on their loved one's condition. Yet they are an invaluable resource for the nursing staff. Family and friends have that one-on-one time, usually for hours, that the facility staff isn't able to provide. The best time for the staff to catch a change in condition is when they assist an elder to get up for the day or help her get into bed.

However, that is when problems occur because the staff member may:

- not be the usual caregiver
- be a caregiver who's not perceptive

- be the caregiver who sees a change but assumes that "everyone already knows"
- be someone with poor communication skills
- be a new nursing assistant or one with little experience

Such a situation places responsibility on the front-line workers who have the least amount of education. Such workers may think of their job primarily in terms of the tasks they have to accomplish. When asked, they usually have the information, but didn't realize they needed to pass it on to the nurse.

That isn't an uncommon problem, and questions naturally arise. For what should the family watch and listen? What is the most effective way to communicate the observation without seeming confrontational or judgmental? Here are four things to notice and also possible guidelines.

1. **Be aware of the elder's pain.** Pain is the most underreported problem in nursing communities. This applies to the general population and even more so for those with dementia. Sometimes the elders can't express their pain in words, so those who know them need to be alert and able to read their body language. Signs of pain in elders with dementia may be increased restlessness, holding a body part, or a sad facial expression. Or it may be a language issue.

One time I walked through a unit for people with dementia. A patient named Edna moved around all the time, so we sat her in a rocker. She rocked for hours at a time, and yelled at anyone who came near her.

We heard her words, but we couldn't understand her language. We didn't even know what language she spoke. During the first two weeks after her arrival, we asked bilingual people to help us. We asked all through the building and we also asked visitors to listen and see if they could identify her language. No one could understand her. Edna had no family to help us communicate.

One day as I walked though the unit, an elderly gentleman, a neighbor of Edna's, had come to visit. He walked over to the nearest nurse and asked, "Don't you know Edna is in pain?" The nurse said no one understood her words.

"She's from Yugoslavia and she's calling out in Serbian, the language of her childhood."

Just to know that information helped us to give her better care. Even more important, we were able to do something to control her pain. Her neighbor came by often, and he also gave us a list of Serbian words she used to express her pain. If only someone on staff had been able to communicate with her, Edna could have been given something to relieve her pain. That's an isolated case, but it reminds us that we have to learn the language of pain, especially when we deal with those with dementia.

Elders with chronic pain should have routine orders for pain medication. Orders for pain medication written "as needed" or PRN are not appropriate in a chronic condition. When the order is PRN for someone with arthritis, that means we have to rely on the nursing assistants to notice that when they bend the elder's knees and observe a grimace, or the joint may be swollen or warm to the touch, the elder is hurting. When elders suffer from any kind of chronic pain, they don't sleep well. Fatigue is another symptom. Or they may not eat well and begin to withdraw.

A nursing assistant is there to assist, and it lays a heavy responsibility on them—for which they're not trained—to observe and communicate to the nurse. That's why the family can be of immense help and support to the staff. When family members observe signs of pain, they can communicate effectively by stating the behavior, area of the body, and provide any history the nurses need.

"I noticed that Mom is rubbing her knees," a daughter may say. "She has had problems with arthritis in the past, and it must be bothering her again." The daughter may have said that after spending hours with her mother. Nurses saw her mother only at brief intervals.

An article in the *Wall Street Journal* of December 4, 2007, written by Lucette Lagnado, stated that Medicaid has spent more money on antipsychotic drugs for Americans than they have on any other class, and that includes antibiotics, AIDS drugs, and medication for high blood pressure. The reason: Some nursing homes use powerful antipsychotic drugs to subdue elders. It keeps the elders quiet, and it adds up the costs for Medicaid. The report said that the staff gave those drugs "to elderly patients to quiet symptoms of Alzheimer's disease and other forms of dementia."

The article also reported that nearly 30 percent of the total nursing-home population receive antipsychotic drugs; far more than needed. "In a practice known as 'off-label' use of prescription drugs, patients can get these powerful medicines whether they are psychotic or not." The article went on to say that 21 percent of nursing home patients who don't have a psychosis diagnosis are on antipsychotic drugs.

Lagnado cited the case of an eighty-four-year-old Alzheimer's patient in a nursing home in Medina, New York, who nervously tapped her foot and rolled her wheelchair around the unit. Her behavior bothered the staff, and they considered it disruptive. They gave her "a powerful antipsychotic drug called Seroquel, a drug approved for schizophrenia and bipolar disorder." The woman had neither. The article focused on the cost of such drugs. Seroquel can cost more than four dollars a pill; the concern must be more for the elder than the cost.

This is where families must be aware of all medication their loved one receives. It's too easy, in some facilities, to give elders a powerful drug to keep them quiet. The drug works, but it is not good nursing care; it is not good humanitarian care. If you are suspicious about medication, ask what the elder receives, why he or she needs it, and who prescribed it.

2. Observe the elder's skin. Skin is the largest organ of the body. In the average person, the skin stretches about two square yards and is about 15 percent of the individual's weight. We consider the skin the first line of defense against environmental factors. Skin is also a barometer of health. We want to be aware of any redness, warmth, or swelling. It is perfectly appropriate for family members or friends to ask the nursing assistant, "Does she have any skin problems?" When elders sit for hours in a wheelchair or are unable to move themselves independently, they may be at risk for their skin to break down because of decreased circulation.

For example, when we brought my uncle Ed to his nursing community, we asked to see what mattresses were available. Uncle Ed had advanced Alzheimer's disease. That meant he would no longer initiate much movement. Because we voiced our concern, the community provided Ed with a special pressure-relieving mattress that kept him comfortable and free of skin breakdown until he died.

A special pressure-relieving or gel cushion is an excellent aid for wheelchair-bound residents. After Mother's stroke, we purchased a pressure-relieving cushion for her wheelchair. That was money well spent for prevention. The pain involved with a skin ulcer can be traumatic and there is also the cost of healing an open area in the skin.

3. **Report any significant change.** The rule of thumb is that a dramatic change in any body system must be reported to the physician immediately. This includes an abrupt change in

- behavior
- difficulty arousing the elder
- high fever
- dizziness or unsteadiness
- sight or hearing
- ability to communicate or speech patterns

- personality
- eating
- difficulty swallowing
- weakness or decreased use of an extremity.

Elders must be watched constantly for anything that appears suddenly and is dramatically different from the norm for that individual.

4. **What to do after the elder falls.** When a family member learns of a fall, the first questions should be:

- "Did anyone see the fall?"
- "Did she hit her head?"
- "Is the person's language indicative of pain?" (A groan, for example.)
- "Are there any outward signs of pain?"

There are many benefits from walking if elders are able to do so. Yet too often families want elders forced into wheelchairs prematurely to keep them "safe" after a fall. Elders want to remain as independent as possible. Even those who are demented but still able to walk can experience opportunities for interaction while "wandering" the community. When wandering, they have opportunities for social interaction, such as when staff personnel greet them by name.

They can remain strong. They may wander, but they also maintain the ability to walk. As an added benefit, it enables them to work up an appetite, breathe deeper, and it supports the process of elimination.

General Guidelines for Families

When you have identified a change in the elder's usual condition:

- Don't hesitate to voice your concern to the nursing staff.
- Identify and talk to staff who may be more pro-active in problem solving.
- Establish yourself as part of the team caring for the elder.
- Be willing to participate as part of the solution.
- Realize that seeing an unaddressed change in condition can be stressful. Try to communicate your concern without becoming overly emotional.
- Pray for your loved one.

Chapter 8

WHO'S ON FIRST?

[Jesus said] "And the King will tell them, 'I assure you, when you did it to one of the least of these my brothers and sisters, you were doing it to me!'"

(Matt. 25:40)

Who are these people who have chosen to serve and take care of the widow in her distress? Following are typical job descriptions.

Certified Nursing Assistant

I read this job description in the *Chicago Tribune* in an article about careers: Nursing Assistants provide routine care such as bathing, dressing, and grooming to elderly, convalescent, or disabled patients at a residential-care facility. Employees in this field require short-term on-the-job training and a general knowledge of medicine, psychology, counseling, and clerical duties. Communication, social perception, and time management skills are also desirable.

Yet this is considered an entry-level job in health care with maybe, but not always, a high school diploma, and about seventy-five hours of training. For many nursing assistants, this was their entry-level position; for others this is what they are doing by default, because it is the best paying job they can get at the moment. But for still others, the solid base of this area of the health care team is the long term *career* nursing assistant.

They are the key people for the family to get to know. They are the day-to-day caregivers who know the current condition and any issues that need to be addressed. They are the caregivers that you want to communicate special needs, likes, and dislikes, so that they can provide the best of care. Even though nursing assistants are probably the lowest paid staff in the organization, they provide 90 percent of the hands-on care.

The term "hands-on" means so much. Many times in a nursing community the elder gets touched only during routine basic care. It will be the caring nursing assistant who notices that the elder looks a little down today. The nursing assistant is the one who speaks words of encouragement, offers a hug or a smile, or pauses a moment to listen.

When I come to visit my mother, my goal is to be part of the team and to straighten the closet, wash my mother's glasses, answer the mail, organize the bedside table and drawers, and do anything else that I can do to help. If I can bring in donuts, a tin of popcorn, or bake something for Mother, I gladly share that with the staff.

For example, when Joseph, one of my mother's favorite assistants, tells me he enjoys sitting with her and watching the DVD of her pictures with her, I know that his time management skills are appropriate.

Chaplain

Some nursing communities are fortunate to have their own chaplain on staff. Becoming acquainted with that individual will be important for the elder. Share the elder's history. Find out what services are offered, such as Bible classes in-house, and what Christian radio stations they receive. On admission, find out how to communicate personal requests.

My dad made it part of his ministry to visit the widows on the anniversary of their husband's death. Those widows, whether living in their homes or a nursing community, waited for his arrival that day, because they knew he would come. Prior to the anniversary of my dad's death, I remind Mother's chaplain of that date so that he is able to schedule time with her. I can't always arrange to be with her on that anniversary, but the comfort of knowing Pastor Paul is there helps our whole family.

Administrator

Administrators usually spend 90 percent of their time reacting, and are lucky to have 10 percent of their time to act. They are responsible for all departments, for the property, for following local, state, and federal guidelines. The administrator sets the pay scales for every department and has to answer to the owner for the entire budget. When the annual state survey is conducted, the administrator assumes the responsibility for the outcome of the survey. The administrator must be licensed by the state, and any judgments found against a nursing facility will also show up on the public record against the administrator's license. You can find this information on the Internet. When there is a dispute with any department, whether it is about environmental, billing, or care issues, the administrator is the final authority.

Medical Director

The medical director is many times a physician with a practice outside the nursing community. The medical director usually has the largest number of patients in the facility. This happens because many times an individual's personal physician will not follow the resident into the nursing community. The residents might have moved from out of state to be closer to children, or they may be without a physician. The facility will assign a physician to them, and it is usually the medical director. The medical director also steps in if for any reason a resident's personal physician can't be reached.

If your elder's own physician will not follow him or her after admittance into the nursing community, the admitting nurse should provide the information so you can know which staff doctor has been assigned.

The attending physician writes orders that direct the care of the elder. The physician's orders cover not only the medications but also treatments, diet guidelines and restrictions, therapies, and laboratory tests. The elder's health care power of attorney should have the physician's phone number so that the family may call the physician directly with concerns.

Director of Nursing

This is a registered nurse who oversees the entire nursing department. This nurse manages and directs all of the programs and systems in the nursing department, such as monitoring residents' weights, skin breakdown, incidents of falls and other injuries, infections, hiring of nursing staff, scheduling of staff, and works closely with the laboratory and pharmacy. Any care issues should be directed to the floor nurse, and if unresolved, taken to the Director of Nursing. In some nursing communities there is an Assistant Director of Nursing who assumes some of the director's roles, but ultimately reports to the Director of Nursing.

Nurses

Every resident has a specific nurse responsible for the elder's care every shift, seven days a week. The nursing assistants report to that nurse any changes in condition, behavior, or issue they have noted during their care. The nurse depends on the reliable report of the nursing assistant. The nurse is responsible for the accuracy of the delivery of care as outlined in the physician's orders. The nurse also assesses elders for risk for falls, risk for skin breakdown, and conducts a current skin assessment of any problem areas. That person also notifies the pharmacy of medication orders and calls the laboratory for any doctor-ordered tests.

The nurse makes arrangements for the labeling of clothes, dentures, glasses, and hearing aids. It's a good idea to inquire about the systems in place for monitoring those pieces of personal property. I recommend having insurance on some items, especially costly hearing aids.

Dietitian

All physicians' diet orders are reviewed by the dietitian. The dietitian also does an evaluation of the nutritional needs of your elder, which is based on height and current weight. Meeting with or communicating with the dietitian about the elder's food preferences, likes, dislikes, and food allergies is of the utmost importance. The nursing assistant's observations of what foods the elder really likes, and what he or she doesn't seem to eat, are communicated to the dietitian. The family can easily help with this communication on admission, as needed, and at quarterly care conferences.

Recreational Therapist/Activity Director

On admission, the activity director completes an assessment of the elder's past and current recreational interests. An activity calendar is posted and it is a good idea to review this calendar and indicate to nursing, as well as activity staff, which activities would really be enjoyed by your elder.

Find ways to be your elder's activity director. When I visit on Sundays, I bring the Sunday paper, and Mother and I go over the television programming for the next week. I make a list of the programs she wants to see and hang it on the wall next to the TV to inform staff. If there is nothing on that appeals to her, I indicate that she would like to see one of her DVDs of her "life story" pictures, or maybe one of the musicals she loves.

Social Services

This is the person who collects all of the personal history of the elder. If your nursing community has only a form that covers where the elder was born, where did she go to school, who she was or is married to, and how many children they have, you need to write your own letter of introduction to the community.

The social services individual serves as a resource for the family by providing information regarding systems and services. Education regarding Do Not Resuscitate orders (DNR) will be communicated through the Social Service Department on admission, and as needed following a change in condition. Information regarding outside services and support organizations, referrals to specialists, Resident's Rights, room changes, and participating in the Plan of Care for the elder are also responsibilities of Social Services.

That person is the individual with whom you should share concerns if your elder seems withdrawn or depressed. Social services usually offers counseling for the elder, as well as the family, with coping problems related to placement, chronic illness, or terminal illness. The Social Service Department can provide Hospice information and make the necessary arrangements.

In my career I have often heard families lament that they have told "everyone" their concern. Then I learned that they had told the nursing assistant numerous times what the concern was, but no one ever passed it on to the appropriate department. Requesting a list of the phone numbers and email addresses of the management team can avoid feelings of frustration through a much more timely response to a concern. However, at times if the family member takes a step back and thinks about how he or she can, as part of the team, help with the issue, it can turn out to be a win-win experience for everyone.

Chapter 9

RESIDENTS' RIGHTS

> For everything there is a season, a time for every activity under heaven. A time to be born and a time to die. A time to plant, and a time to harvest.
>
> (Eccl. 3:1-2)

State laws legislate the Residents' Bill of Rights that provides guidelines to facility employees to provide effective and personal care. The bill of rights also explains for residents and families the responsibility they share in making certain their needs have been attended to and that their wishes have been honored.

The Right to Advanced Directives

On admission to a nursing community, residents or their designated surrogate decision maker have to make choices about medical treatments and document them through the Right to Advanced Directives. To avoid potential future misunderstandings, families need to be clear among themselves what they want. The staff is mandated to support the decisions made by the surrogate. If they are unable to support the decision, they shouldn't be involved in the care of that individual.

The inability to support the decision of the family could be as simple as the case of an elderly woman who lives in the community for several years and becomes a favorite of the staff. The woman has a major stroke, and there is no hope for her recovery. The family's decision was made in the past (based on the knowledge of the wishes of the woman, which she had voiced over a lifetime) not to put in a feeding tube. Because of her deep emotional attachment, one staff member can't allow the woman to die naturally. She becomes judgmental of the family and especially of the individual carrying the Health Care Power of Attorney.

That staff member should not have been involved. It is not her right to choose whether to use a feeding tube. Her attitude can confuse the family and cause alienation. During difficult times, families need support, not judgmental attitudes or attempts to override the expressed wishes of the family and the elder.

Those who hold the Health Care Power of Attorney need to be diligent in checking the elder's chart that current Do Not Resuscitate forms (DNR) are present. If the elder has gone out to the hospital, chances are that the original DNR form went with the elder and was not returned. Members of support staff do not usually honor photocopies.

Dying elders and their families have unique needs for respectful, responsive care. The family, as well as the elder, deserves to receive support during the elder's final days. When there is a terminal illness, the nursing community can contact a Hospice provider the family has chosen to use. (Before you need their service, it's wise to interview several hospice representatives to find out the services they offer.)

The Right to Privacy and Confidentiality

In a nursing community the staff is allowed access only to information necessary to do their job. The housekeepers may need to know that the elder has allergies so they won't use aerosol products in the room, but they don't need to know that the elder has cancer.

If done properly, all employees will sign a form to protect health care information. Nursing communities should follow the Health Insurance Portability and Accountability Act (HIPPA compliance). The nursing community should have a HIPPA officer and provide their name to new families. The family needs to report violations of privacy to the facility HIPPA officer as well as the administrator.

This sounds obvious, and yet, even in small ways, the right of privacy is sometimes violated. For example, staff members may give private information in a public area when they call out, "Has Mary had a BM today?" or "Does Bob still have diarrhea?" They are guilty of violating elders' confidentiality. Suppose family members, who are regular visitors, inquire why they haven't seen a familiar face recently. A staff member says, "Oh, Ethel had a stroke last week and isn't doing well." Such conversations occur all too frequently in a nursing community and violate an elder's right to privacy. The staff member can respond with a simple "I'm sorry but we aren't able to give out health care information."

Many times staff members have become too casual and accustomed to sharing information. Receiving input from visitors who have been rightly surprised and offended by this form of interaction can make staff more aware of their casual conversation.

Be aware that if an elder is in a facility or a unit known for a particular condition such as Alzheimer's, just by giving out information such as the name of one of their residents, staff are divulging medical information.

When appropriate, however, the family may ask staff to share the elder's change of condition with other residents. Many times someone who has lived with them for years, and possibly eaten at their table, just disappears, and the residents want to know what happened.

The Right to Respectful Treatment

The staff should treat elders in a courteous and prompt manner. Visitors may become aware of staff talking down to an elder, or speaking in a manner that is demeaning or scolding. They should report such behavior.

For instance, one Sunday when I visited my mother in her room, she told me that during the past week she had come into her room and the facility cat—an animal to which she was highly allergic—was on her bed. As soon as she spotted the cat, she chased it from her room.

The housekeeper, who was cleaning the bathroom, came out, and shook her index finger into my then eighty-two-year-old mother's face. "Verona, don't you yell at that cat. She is old!"

Her words shocked me. *Every* staff member needs to be aware of what it means to be respectful to their elders.

The Right to Communication

Elders in a nursing community have the right to receive personal phone calls, their mail, visitors, and other communication as long as it doesn't affect their treatment. That statement sounds obvious, but it's not always easy to accomplish.

Reaching Mother by phone became problematic. When Dad was alive he answered the phone and passed it on to Mother. With Dad gone, we had to come up with a plan, because she wouldn't answer the phone. We worked through that, and she agreed to answer. We had a phone put on her nightstand; that didn't work because she couldn't reach it. We decided that a portable phone would be the answer. However, the only outlet to charge the phone that was also convenient to the telephone hookup could be reached only by staff. We knew we couldn't expect the staff to remember to put the phone on the charger at night and give it to her to carry in her purse the next day. Because of the floating of staff and staff turnover it was impossible to notify everyone, and even if we could, we knew it wouldn't work.

We thought the answer was a phone on a bedside table; however, the facility didn't have a bedside table available.

We bought a bedside table at a home health care drug store. We purchased a simple touchtone phone with no fancy buttons to push. She only had to pick up the receiver and say hello.

We installed the phone with an extra-long cord to run behind the furniture and used Velcro to fasten it to her bedside table. After that, whenever she was in bed, the phone was within her reach. This worked out well most of the time. When we were unable to reach Mother in the evenings, we knew the reason: The nursing assistant who put her to bed had forgotten to put the table back in place.

The Right to Make Informed Decisions

Elders, as well as families or other designated persons, have the right to full explanation of diagnosis, proposed treatment, and procedures, given in terms that are easily understood. They have the right to have an "interpreter" present to help them understand pertinent information. The explanation should include the benefits of the treatment, the risks involved, possible significant complications, and the probable outcome of the treatment as well as alternative treatments.

Elders and their representatives have the right to review any records that pertain to their healthcare.

The Right to Participate in All Aspects of Healthcare

Elders or their surrogate decision makers have the right to be involved in all choices about their plan of care. They should be made aware when the interdisciplinary team will meet to discuss the elder's care plan *and should be included as part of the team.* Special considerations for the rights of the cognitively impaired include:

- humane, appropriate treatment
- protection from harm in the treatment setting
- freedom from unnecessary or excessive medication
- freedom from physical restraint and isolation, except in well-defined emergency
- freedom from retaliation

The Right to Impartial Access to Care

Residents have the right to receive impartial access to healthcare regardless of race, national origin, age, creed, sex, or source of payment.

Knowledge of Rights and Responsibilities in Receiving Care

Residents and their families have the right to be informed of facility policies and practices that relate to resident care, treatment, and responsibilities, *including financial responsibilities.*

One of the big surprises for a family is the cost of everyday supplies. Before admitting an elder, family members need to ask, "What is included in the room rate?" If the nursing staff makes additional charges for every box of tissue and every bag of incontinent supplies, the cost will be much more than families anticipated.

Before you choose a nursing community, request a copy of their Resident's Rights. Read it carefully before you make your final decision.

Chapter 10

WHAT IF IT'S ALZHEIMER'S DISEASE?

> [God says] "Don't be afraid, for I am with you. Don't be discouraged, for I am your God. I will strengthen you and help you. I will hold you up with my victorious right hand."
>
> (Isa. 41:10)

It was a winter's afternoon, and I felt the need for a little sugar rush to get me through the rest of the day. I went down to the vending area in the employee cafeteria. There sat the son of one of our elders, who was a frequent visitor. I asked if he was coming or going.

"I'm trying to come," he said.

It seemed as though every time he visited, he had to go to the cafeteria for a few minutes and emotionally ready himself for the visit with his mother, whom he loved dearly. "She's in the late stage of Alzheimer's disease and no longer recognizes me," he said. It was obvious that hurt him deeply.

Many books have been written about the long, painful loss of a person to Alzheimer's disease. But while that is certainly true, it is also true that during this time of loss the ongoing life of the person continues. Visiting with a person afflicted with Alzheimer's disease becomes more of a connection than a "visit." Let's look at three kinds of memory.

1. **Declarative Memory**
   When someone is first diagnosed with Alzheimer's disease the focus is on the *declarative memory* that is lost. Declarative memory is the ability to consciously remember recent and remote events, mathematical formulas, vocabulary, and facts—such as the ability to answer, "What did you do today?" or, "Where did you park the car?"

2. **Procedural Memory**
   Procedural memory, also called *non-declarative memory*, means to learn and remember by doing. That includes repetitive activity, habits, motor learning, and emotional memory. That body or muscle memory is referred to when people say that once you learn to ride a bike, you can always ride a bike.

   Non-declarative, or procedural memory, in an individual with Alzheimer's disease, is preserved long after declarative memory is lost.

3. **Emotional Memory**
   Emotional memory can involve family traditions remembered through sight, smells, and hearing.

> Decorating the elder's room for the Christmas holidays, singing Christmas carols, bringing in cookies, and reading the Nativity Story from Luke 2 are things that tap into that emotional memory bank.

I have seen memory still demonstrated into what is known as the late stage of Alzheimer's disease. One such woman was Lilly. She had been a classical pianist. She wandered aimlessly from room to room in the nursing community. Lilly was non-verbal, unable to recognize family, staff, or even herself in a mirror. But if, in her wandering, she happened upon the piano, she sat down and her hands hit those long-practiced keys, and her body remembered the moves. For a few minutes, Lilly could play the most extraordinarily beautiful music. Then she would get up and move along again as if the moment had never occurred.

We know that no two people are exactly alike, and that Alzheimer's disease affects people differently, depending on what area of the brain is most affected. The loss of function usually follows a pattern. Most elders lose abilities in the reverse order that they gained the ability.

Take the ability to dress themselves. Children learn first to put on simple items such as shirt and pants. The child progresses to being able to button, put on socks and shoes, and later to tie her shoes. For a long time she may put on shorts with a winter sweater before learning that certain things go together. She progresses to the point where she learns the necessity of changing and wearing clean clothes. And eventually she learns about the right season, occasion, or temperature for which she is dressing.

Elders with Alzheimer's disease will lose the *last learned ability first*. They will be unable to dress correctly for the season or temperature. So you may see elders in summer with a winter coat and hat on that they insist on wearing. They are still able to follow through with the long practiced skills of putting on clothes correctly, but they can no longer choose appropriately.

The most troublesome ability for elders with Alzheimer's disease is the issue of continence. Small children will become continent of bowels before urine. They progress to be able to toilet themselves and finally to provide for their own hygiene. So also, the elder losing the skills in the reverse order no longer provides adequate bathroom hygiene. Then he has trouble making it to the bathroom in time, or finds the bathroom, but becomes incontinent of urine and finally bowels. Knowing this progression of the disease can aid family members in their expectations of the elder.

When visiting, plan to do an activity together. Do that instead of talking when the elder can no longer remember the events or facts being discussed. Doing an activity together, especially an activity that would involve long or over-practiced movements, can tap into that procedural memory and create a connection.

With supervision, a woman who loved to knit may be able once again to hold those knitting needles and enjoy holding balls of different types of yarn. A man who loved to fish may enjoy a fishing box with harmless lures to hold.

Here are a few activity suggestions:

- Clip coupons.
- Toss a ball.
- Color a picture.
- Bring in a pet.
- Cut pictures out of greeting cards.
- Sing. (Many elders who are no longer able to talk can sing well-known songs, such as "Jesus Loves Me" or "Amazing Grace.")
- Put a simple puzzle together.
- Sew sewing cards.
- Give the elder a manicure.
- Mold with Play Doh.
- Look at pictures.
- Trace something.
- Bring in a seasonal activity from a craft store.

As the disease progresses, the elder will exhibit a progressively lower stress threshold. Try to visit in a quiet area and not in the middle of a noisy dining room full of distractions.

Even elders in the late stage of dementia can usually recognize someone as a friend. Make direct eye contact, get on the same level as the elder, and speak the person's name and smile while you communicate. Even something as simple as touching the elders' hands while you talk can bring his or her attention right to the speaker.

While communicating, incorporate as many senses as you can: hearing, seeing, and touching will make a connection even in the very late stages of the disease. Although the elder may no longer recognize you as a spouse or child, your body language will communicate to the elder that she knows you.

When visiting, avoid the use of pronouns. Be very literal, and speak using nouns. When speaking about people, identify them by name. Instead of saying, "He is parking the car," say, "Your brother, Bob, is parking the car."

The sound of laughter can be comforting. My dad told me once that when he was going in for his heart surgery he remembered coming out of the effects of the anesthesia and hearing us all there, and we were laughing. That comforted him. When my sister and I sit with Mother and the three of us laugh, many visitors stop us and tell us how the sound of that laughter helped them.

The sound of the human voice comforts a baby, and so also can comfort the elder. Reading a favorite book, poem, or passages from the Bible to the elder can provide the stimulation and comfort of the voice.

Don't ask open-ended questions of the elder. "What did you have for lunch today?" Being unable to recall such information can cause stress for the elder.

If the elder is speaking in nonsensical words, don't pretend to understand. Or if the elder voices confused thoughts such as, "My mother is coming to pick me up," don't correct the error. Instead, interact with something non-related.

Use the power of touch when you visit. Hold a hand and squeeze it while you speak, or give a gentle kiss. Such gestures can be very reassuring. Use hand lotion and provide a hand massage as a wonderful form of connection. Brush the elder's hair or give hugs to make the elder feel secure.

Watch sensory videos or DVDs, because they can be relaxing, especially those with the sounds of nature. Turn on soft music and touch the elder gently, because that provides companionship and a sense of belonging.

When elders are no longer able to communicate verbally, they can still connect with the world through their senses. Elders with Alzheimer's disease can also continue to connect emotionally. They still appreciate a hug, a smile, a handshake, soft words, and a loving look.

They can still find peace, security, and companionship by seeing family members, or by hearing familiar hymns or Scripture passages. The voices of their loved ones, or the smell of a familiar fragrance or a favorite food can stimulate them. They can respond to the touch of a baby, a loved pet, and holding someone's hand. Some have found that providing warm, cuddly toys for the elders is helpful.

Chapter 11

THE CHRISTIAN'S JOY

> But the angel reassured [the shepherds], "Don't be afraid!" he said, "I bring you good news that will bring great joy to all people. The Savior—yes, the Messiah, the Lord—has been born today in Bethlehem, the city of David!"
>
> (Luke 2:10-11)

Sunday afternoons are the times I spend with Mother. We eat lunch together, visit, and discuss issues from the previous week. We read any mail received during the week. I fuss about the room with any organizational tasks that need to be done. We discuss her current health issues and concerns. We may play cards, or if it is close to a holiday season, we sing hymns of the season. I read aloud for quite a long time, until I sense she is beginning to tire. Mother tells anyone that her favorite time of the week is when I come and read to her.

I read from many Christian authors, but the theme is always the same. She wants me to read about heaven. Mother has, like many elders, an unquenchable thirst for education and discussion about heaven. She wants to talk about what it looks like, what we will do there, what we will eat, who will be there, will we know each other? Fortunately, there are authors who have devoted time to this subject. We enjoy Joni Eareckson Tada, Anne Graham Lotz, Randy Alcorn's *Heaven*, and *90 Minutes in Heaven* by Don Piper with Cecil Murphey. Piper and Murphey also wrote *Heaven Is Real*. Those authors have searched the scriptures for us. Those books have been such a blessing to us, stimulating conversations with Mother that I would not otherwise have had.

I am only there on Sunday afternoons. While I am there I can create an atmosphere of support, concern, mental stimulation, and then I'm gone. Who or what can fill the void of all of those hours in a day? Yes, the staff are there, but they are task oriented. Nurses have those pills to pass and nursing assistants have their duties. Activity staff are concerned with the big picture of creating meaningful programming for every elder.

Who or what is there to fill that empty void for Mother? I asked that question for several days, and then I knew the answer: Christian radio! Christian radio brings comfort, Bible study, music, and news. It provides a positive atmosphere and brings joy. She listens to local, national, and world news that not only keeps her informed, but also empowers her and gives her purpose and desire to live. For example, when Mother hears of an accident on the interstate and the announcer reminds the audience that there are people out there who need prayer, that is something she can do. She feels empowered and useful.

When Mother hears about issues of national debate, she is not only informed, but continues to be part of society by being able to join in conversations. She is empowered as she prays for the president, members of Congress, or the judiciary.

When there are major catastrophes. Mother participates by joining her prayers with other Christians thousands of miles away. When Christians are persecuted in the name of Jesus Christ, she can be part of the solution through prayer. Because of their life experience, older Christians have had a personal history with the power of prayer, and Christian radio gives them the opportunity to exercise that muscle and keep it strong.

Christian radio creates an atmosphere in Mother's room that cannot help but impact the staff when they are there providing care. The staff member seems to be more patient, kinder, and more understanding when the message of the love of Christ is in that room through the airwaves.

Not only are the staff not as likely to engage in inappropriate language or conversation, but there is no way to know what message they receive while providing routine care. Mother has had many opportunities to witness in conversations with staff while they do the most basic of care. When a message is being shared over the airwaves and the caregiver expresses a question, Mother is able to explain.

Christian radio supports and, most of all, triggers the kind of reminiscing that brings joy and comfort to elders.

We live much of our lives inside our minds. Memories are stored in many different areas of our brains under different triggers. Mother can't hear "How Great Thou Art" without thinking of Dad, because that was his favorite hymn.

Listening to the radio keeps her in the season and helps her to pass the long nights when she is unable to sleep. One day when I visited, Mother said she had awakened during the night and the most beautiful music was playing, and she thought, *This must be just like heaven.* As I stared at the joy on Mother's face, it made me grateful to the nursing assistant who had turned on the radio that night.

Nursing community staff are so used to taking residents to their rooms and turning on the TV without regard for what is on. Few residents express interest in anything on television, other than re-runs of the weekly *Lawrence Welk Show, Wheel of Fortune*, or an old familiar movie. The usual array of crime drama, soap operas, talk shows, and court TV may contribute to feelings of depression and helplessness. Published studies on young children have shown the detrimental effects of these kinds of programming. I believe they're also detrimental to elders

Having the staff know that, when Verona is in her room and going to bed she listens to her radio station, makes a statement to the staff of who Verona is. I believe they can see her Christ-like witness as she faces difficult days and sometimes a difficult life. Hearing Christian radio supports her faith and provides a sense of continuity amid the changes she faces, and gives her peace.

No amount of money, power, or prestige could provide the peace, comfort, contentment, and pure joy Mother is able to receive every hour of every day from the dedicated Christian speakers and musicians coming from that dear little black box on her nightstand. I wish that every elder in a nursing community could have access to Christian radio, because it has the power to inform, comfort, and keep them strong in their faith, until they "take Jesus' hand."

Chapter 12

LET GO AND LET GOD

> Don't worry about anything; instead, pray about everything. Tell God what you need, and thank him for all he has done.
>
> (Phil. 4:6)

Dad taught me how to pray. When I was a young child, Dad taught me to "make going to God a part of your daily life." He said I could go anytime, anywhere, with anything and everything. Dad told me that Jesus taught us how to ask: " . . . and when you ask, do it in Jesus' name." He said, "Always end with the words, 'Thy will be done,' because you don't know what is best for you. Remember that God's time is always right."

These were exactly the prayers we needed when Dad went through his journey with Alzheimer's disease. We started where most families start—the awareness that Dad was no longer safe to drive his car. "How can we get him off the road?" we asked each other.

Mother had already had a stroke and lived in a nursing community. The plan was to move her to a place where Dad could also have an apartment and no longer had to drive to see her. That plan worked out very well, and soon after the move, we got rid of the car.

Dad recruited a little band of volunteers on whom he called when he needed transportation. Although the loss of his independence was a serious adjustment for him, he joked that it took a village to get him to church, the Bible class that he still taught at another nursing community, his barber, the grocery store, and the doctors. Dad wasn't shy about asking for help. (After his death, those volunteers introduced themselves to us at the funeral as Dad's drivers. Each told us how much he or she had enjoyed the time spent with him.)

After the move to the nursing community, Dad's condition deteriorated, and we faced ongoing issues during the next two years. The fire he started in the kitchen was the first problem. (We had to have his stove turned off.) When we took him to the store we realized that he could no longer identify money. He made mistakes with his medication, and we had to have a nurse come in and put his pills together and eventually monitor his taking them.

He no longer took care of his apartment, so that increased the amount of assistance the facility provided. Eventually the staff did the laundry, cleaning, and even the dishes that he had enjoyed washing himself. Because of all the assistance he received, he had many normal days. But sometimes there was a glitch, like the time he spent all day in his apartment because he couldn't find his false teeth.

At every change and decline we had to remember to "Let go and let God." It wasn't always easy, and sometimes we shed private tears, but we knew we had to let go of the situation and trust God to take care of Dad.

Letting go didn't mean not acting on behalf of the elder. As changes occurred, we—and Dad—made adjustments. But the choice was either to hold on to the past, deny the seriousness of the situation, or get angry. Instead we decided to release him to God—to let go and let God take care of him. As much as we would have welcomed the opportunity to have everything stay the same, our denial and anger would have intensified the burden of his losses for Dad. Praying, "Not my will but thy will be done," gave us immense peace during those times.

The most troubling loss for Dad was his word-finding skills. He lost the word *microwave*, and for six months before he died he called it the *chiropractor*. When he voiced concern over his lost words, Mother would say, "You have so many words, more than most people. You can afford to lose a few." Sometimes he laughed.

Even during that time of loss, he continued to gravitate to people, and they moved toward him. Whenever I went to visit, people came up to him in the dining room, or greeted him when they passed us in the hall. Whether they were other residents or staff members, Dad knew them. He didn't remember their names, but he knew their "story." Dad had a way of lighting up when he saw anyone coming and acted as if talking to each one was the high point of his day. Everyone seemed to have spent some time with him, and he knew them.

Most families who go through the Alzheimer's journey encounter levels of grief, such as denial, anger, bargaining, and depression. I have known families who wanted to deny what was right in front of their faces. "He doesn't have Alzheimer's." Or, they'll say, "He'll remember again in time."

They just didn't want to see the change in their loved one, and so they didn't. For them, something else or someone else was the problem. "It just can't be the aging process or any disease." That type of thinking makes it a lonely journey for the elder. The family members spewed out their anger on the staff because they came in and Mom's roommate was wearing Mom's best sweater. The family member's anger becomes misplaced, and the elder becomes a catalyst for the struggle between staff and family. The end result is usually a family member who starts to visit less and less and says things such as, "It really doesn't matter anymore. Mom doesn't even know me."

Those levels of grief were never Dad's experience or focus. For Dad, his faith was in the resilience he demonstrated every day despite each loss. Dad talked about his progressive failings, but always in the light of the faith that put everything into perspective. It wasn't the minutia of the day that interested him. It was the people he came into contact with, and he shared his Easter joy with them.

God's Timing Is Always Right

We lost Dad in March of 2005, after a massive stroke. In the emergency room, as Dad slipped deeper and deeper into a coma and could no longer identify what he heard or what he saw, he prayed as long as he could talk. The last two words he ever spoke were *Jesus* and *Heaven*.

As Mother told everyone in the nursing community, she "didn't want a pity party." We voiced to everyone our total contentment in the fact that Dad had been taken before he had to experience the end stages of Alzheimer's disease.

At the luncheon following the funeral, it amazed us that everyone in attendance knew so much about him. They knew about his lifelong love affair with chocolate. Almost everyone who had come in contact with him knew his favorite sports and favorite teams. His love of interesting neckties and his tie collection was legendary.

In the months that followed his death, I realized the comfort that could follow a loss by trying to emulate the qualities I had admired in my father. And in some ways, I tried to become more like Dad. I started to share more of myself with co-workers and friends the way that Dad had. I made an effort to be more attentive to others while they told me about their problems. I thought of the times when Dad talked to people and he was totally in the moment and really with them. Sharing my faith with others seemed to come up more frequently in conversations, just as it had with Dad.

Many examples are in the news of people who have turned pain into purpose. The individuals who start charitable organizations usually do so after a serious loss. That is true with people who march to honor the memory of a loved one, with marches for breast cancer, Parkinson's, and Alzheimer's disease. I've tried to get more involved and do something for others who have to learn how to let go.

As I write this book, Mother is failing. Some days it is more obvious than others. She tells us that one day she will slip away to heaven. While she is still here I am starting to get ready. I work on those relationships and support systems that I will need later on. I don't spend time on anticipatory grief, not when I can still help.

While no one has ever accused me of being artistic, I have started taking drawing classes and enjoy them. When Mother is gone, I will fill my Sunday afternoons with drawing at my kitchen table, while listening to Christian radio just as Mother used to do. I will continue to read about heaven to elders in nursing communities. I will picture Mother in heaven, doing all of the things that she and I talked about and she was looking forward to. For right now, when I pray for Mother, I know who is in control, and that God's timing is always right.

> God says, "But those who trust in the Lord will find new strength. They will soar high on wings like eagles. They will run and not grow weary. They will walk and not faint."
>
> (Isa. 40:31)

Printed in the United States
123806LV00005B/15/P

9 781414 112077